Best Insomnia Remedies

"You don't need drugs to help you sleep anymore."

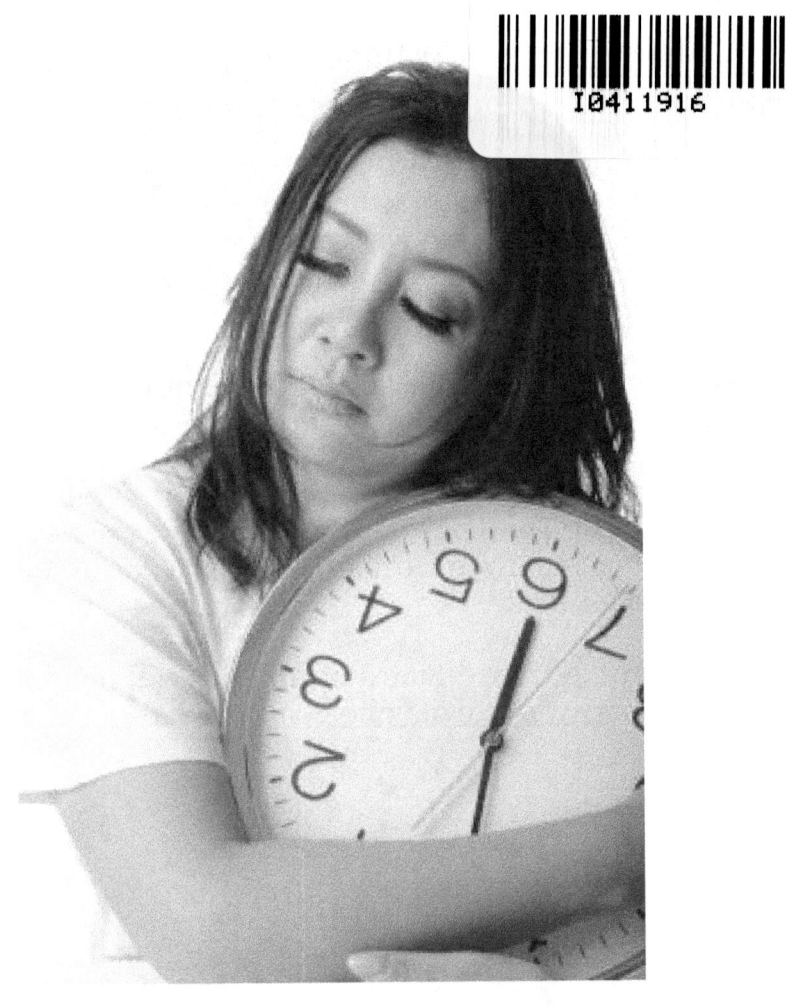

By Rudy S. Silva, Natural Nutritionist

The Best Insomnia Remedies © 2015 by Rudy Silva

ISBN-13: 978-1508800972

ISBN-10: 1508800979

Printed in the United States of America All images provided by: http://www.freedigitalphotos.net

Table of Contents

Ch1: Introduction – Is Insomnia Ruining Your Life

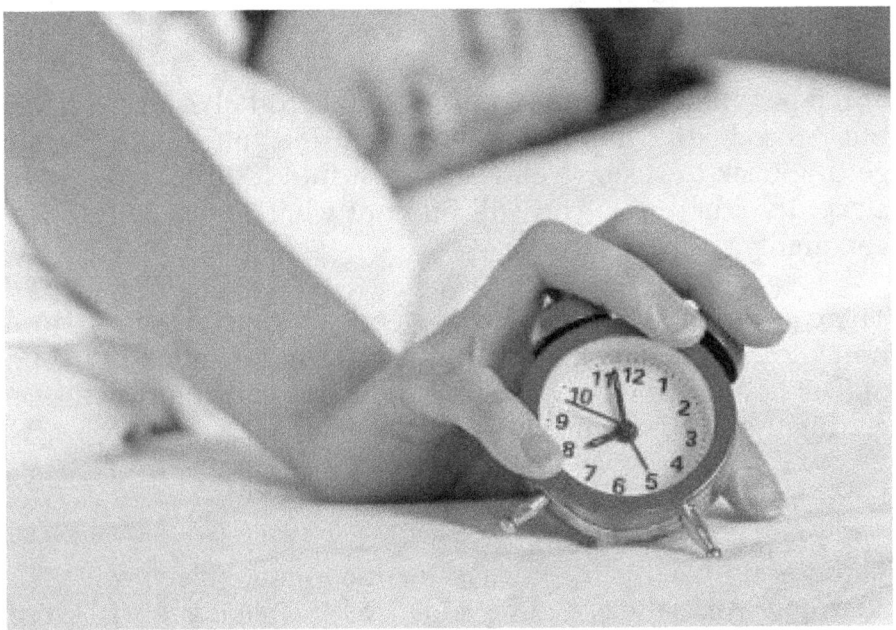

Get one of the best kindle books *free* by **clicking here.**

Stop Insomnia Now

Rudy Silva, Natural Nutritionist here to help you get the best sleep you can get, using natural remedies. I have been helping clients find better health for the last 17 years, and have written many books on natural remedies.

When you sleep, you give your body a chance to rest, sleep, repair, rejuvenate, and detoxify. When this happens, you feel alert and ready to go in the morning. If you have insomnia, whether mild or severe, you disrupt all of these sleep functions.

You can expect to have a better and more energetic life, when you get the right amount of sleep.

If you have difficulty sleeping, there is a likely chance that it relates to anxiety coming from unresolved daily or past issues. There can be other issues that cause sleeplessness and these will also be covered.

Some people with insomnia may be able to fall asleep quickly but wake in the middle of the night and have a hard time getting back to sleep. Yet, others just find it difficult to get to sleep. In either case, you will find out what you need to do to get quality sleep.

There are many ways to get the sleep you need, using natural remedies. This book gives you this information and at the end of this book, will have a chapter on a step by step process on getting the sleep you need.

Drugs for Insomnia?

There is no need to use drugs for insomnia, since with their continually use they become addictive and interfere with your natural sleep cycles. Eventually, these drugs will cause insomnia and have other unwanted side effects.

If you have insomnia, you need to take action right away, since not getting the right amount of sleep is a matter of how long and how well you live.

Insomnia is a condition that is underestimated in the damage it can do to your health. Without the 6+ to 8+ hours sleep that you need, you become more likely to suffer from different ailments and diseases. If you have insomnia, this is one condition you can eliminate and develop feeling of well-being within days or weeks.

In this sleep better book, you will find the foods, natural remedies, supplements and lifestyles that will help you eliminate your insomnia. There is not a lot of fluff here, so you will be able to get started right away on getting yourself back to normal.

The amount of actual sleep needed is different for everyone. The number of hours that you need is based on your age, your daily activities, your health, and your anxieties.

If you suffer from chronic insomnia, your body will make sure you sleep either through dream or hallucination moments.

Ativan for Insomnia

One of the most popular drugs used for sleep is called Ativan (lorazepam.) At their website, WebMD says, "This medication is used to treat anxiety. Lorazepam belongs to a class of drugs known as benzodiazepines which act on the brain and nerves (central nervous system) to produce a calming effect. This drug works by enhancing the effects of a certain natural chemical in the body (GABA)."

This drug is also recommended by doctors for people who have insomnia.
There are over a hundred different drugs and over-the-counter medications available for stress, anxiety, and sleep that you can get, from your doctor or drug store. All have some side effects and in this book, it is recommended that you not use the drug aids. Not only do they have side effects, but they interfere with your natural sleep and body cycles.

Dr. Whitaker, M.D. talks about drugs in his book called Dr. Whitaker's Guide to Natural Healing.

"These drugs [benzodiazepines, Halcion, Ligrium and Valium] can create a vicious cycle in the patient's life. The patient takes the drug to induce sleep. This causes further disruption of

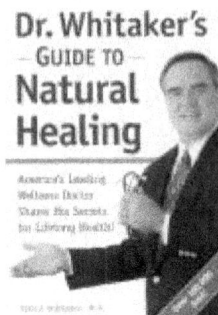

Dr. Whitaker's
GUIDE TO
Natural
Healing

normal sleep by suppressing REM (rapid eye movement) sleep. It is during REM sleep that repair and rejuvenate processes take place. REM sleep is also when we dream... When a patient tries to withdraw from long-term use of benzodiazepines, REM sleep increases. Nightmares and further sleep disturbances are added to other withdrawal symptoms."

Keep in mind that if you have insomnia, you should check with your doctor to make sure you don't and any other medical condition that is causing it.

Ch2: How You Get Insomnia Problems

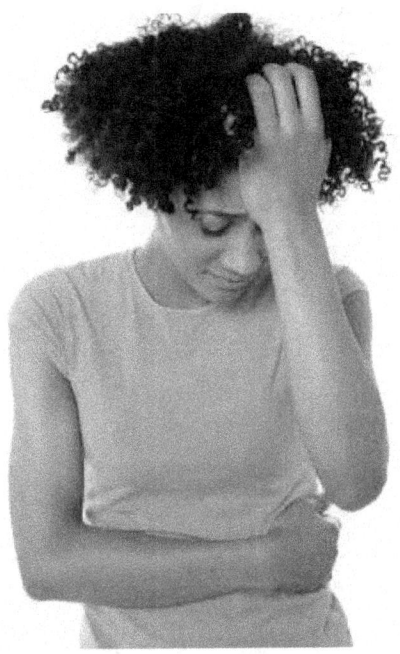

In this chapter, you will discover what cause insomnia and why you are afflicted with this condition.

Sleep

Eight to nine hours of sleep are typically what most people need to maintain a healthy body. When you don't get the sleep, you need, your body produces excess hormones to compensate for this.

During the night, your body is busy digestion, repairing, rebuilding, and detoxifying your body. As you sleep, every hour each organ has it turn in rejuvenating and detoxifying itself.

It's best to get to bed early and get the sleep your body needs.

When you toss and turn and wake frequently at night, you are not getting the rest you need.

Insomnia

Insomnia is a condition where when you wake up you feel like you have not had enough sleep and perhaps have missed out on 2 to 3 hours of sleep. If you experience insomnia for a while, you may exhibit,

- fatigue

- lack of concentration

- irritability

- anxiety

- increase weight

- insulin resistant

- increase blood pressure

The reason that lack of sleep is so critical is that it increases your blood levels of two hormones – cortisol and ACTH. These hormones are related to other chemicals, which are inflammatory and cause degenerative diseases such as,

- Alzheimer's

- Osteoporosis

- Neurodegenerative disorders

- Cardiovascular disease

- Rheumatoid arthritis

- Cancer

So, you want to make sure you get good sleep, unless you want to be predisposed to these and other deadly diseases.

Insomnia

The actual cause of your insomnia is not a simple medical condition. Sleep issues arise from a multitude of problems that cascade throughout your body. But, the real causes of insomnia can arise when you,

1. Have a hormonal imbalance
2. Have stress, anxiety, or depression
3. Hypoglycemia
4. Nutritional deficiencies
5. Illnesses such as lung or heart disease
6. Over active mind
7. Need for recreational or prescription
8. Excess use of caffeine, tobacco, or alcohol
9. Are obese

Hormonal Imbalance

Your sleep is controlled by your brain hypothalamus. It controls the amount of cortisol released from your adrenal gland. Cortisol is release when you are in a state of stress, anxiety, or a threatening situation. This cortisol promotes your pancreas to release glucagon which turns into sugar in your blood. The sugar is used by your brain and muscles as energy to deal with the impending danger or stress.

The problem here is that your body was not built to release cortisol everyday to deal with work stress or other family or friend induced stress. The result of all this stress eventually leads to adrenal burnout, where not enough glucagon is released into your blood to keep your body's energy up. This results in low blood sugar, which has a big impact on your health and typically results in poor quality sleep.

When it's time to go to sleep you may still have high levels of cortisol preventing your from falling asleep quickly. After you fall asleep, your cortisol may drop too low causing you to wake up at night.

Here's what you can expect with adrenal burnout:
- frequently feel irritable

- have difficulty getting along with people or partner

- blood sugar is often low

- you crave sweets

- have frequent colds, sore throats, and infections

- have allergies

- have body aches

- frequently become overwhelm with stress

- develop insulin resistance

- develop heart problems

When you have adrenal burnout, you affect the natural release of glucagon, which gives your hypothalamus the energy and the rest of your body the energy it needs to function naturally.

Anxiety and Insomnia

One of the main reason you may have insomnia is because of anxiety, stress, and depression. If your job that requires a lot of detailed work, and you bring your job home, this can lead to insomnia.

In the book, The Natural Healing and Nutrition, 1990, written by the Staff of Rodale Press, they state, " 'We all need sleep, but we all don't need the same amount," says Ernest Hartmann, M. D., a sleep researcher for 25 years and director of two sleep-disorder centers in Boston. "A lot depends on your personality and what kind of life you lead." People who get along on less sleep tend to be very busy people who are happy with their lives.

Whether or not they're happy, executives tend to get less Sleep — not always by choice. In fact, they even have their own brand of executive insomnia, one of the 120 sleep disorders recognized by the Association of Sleep Disorders Centers in Rochester, Minnesota. Called fibrositis, it is common among intense perfectionists, especially women between 25 and 50, who suffer from shallow sleep because the wake center of their brain remains active."

When you lack sleep it seems to have more of a psychological effect. Daniel Wagner, M.D. , of the Sleep-Wake Center of Cornell University Medical Center, says, "An acute lack of sleep doesn't affect your physical performance, but it does affect your attitude. Not getting enough sleep induces a kind of pessimism. Outside observers probably wouldn't notice this, but you would. You tend to be more critical of yourself, when you don't sleep enough."

Doing work activities just before bedtime, such as budget, checkbook, work projects, can affect your sleep. You need to wind down in preparation for sleep.

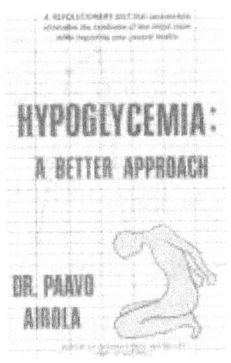

Hypoglycemia

In his book about hypoglycemia, Dr. Paavo Airola reports on Dr. Salzer's finding, "Here is Dr. Salzer's list of the most common symptoms of low blood sugar, based on his questioning of over three hundred hypoglycemic patients whom he had tested. The symptoms are listed along with the percentage of patents complaining of them.

- Exhaustion 67%

- Depression 60%

- Insomnia 50%

- Anxiety 50%

Age

As you age, you need less sleep. Around 50-plus years, you might only need 6 or so hours. And, during this time you might wake up more frequently. But, babies need about 16 hours of sleep.

Body Pains and Twitching

If you experience body twitching and pain in the legs (Restless Legs Syndrome, RLS) at night, this can cause you to lose sleep. Movement in your body at night can prevent you from getting deep sleep, and you wake up tired and sleepy.

This twitching or pain can be related to an acid body. When you have too much acid in your muscle tissue, you can experience pain in various body muscles and typically at night you will have it your calves or big toe.

Any type of body pain can keep you from getting a good night sleep.

Acid Reflux

When you get acid reflux at night, it can raise your body temperature and prevent you from getting deep sleep. Don't use any medication for this issue, since medication for acid reflux is additive. Instead use ¼ teaspoon of baking soda in 6 oz. of water, just before bedtime. This will reduce your stomach acid, but the best solution is to start eating an alkaline diet.

Miscellaneous Causes for Insomnia

- Too much sleep or oversleeping can affect your sleeping patterns. Aim for the amount of sleep that feels right for you and leaves you feeling refreshed and energized.

- Drinking too many caffeinated drinks (coffee, sodas, energy drinks, and some herbal teas) is one way to bring on a case of insomnia because it is a stimulant to the body. Limit your coffee drinking to 3 or 4 cups per day or less.

- You may think that using alcohol to relax and sleep is helping you, but the truth is that it disrupts your brain waves making it hard to fall asleep. And, the next day you may feel tired and have low energy.

- Sleeping in a noisy area or near where noise can be heard. In this case, it may be helpful to invest in a good pair of earplugs, which can give you some sound relief.

- Going to sleep hungry can contribute to sleep disturbances. Eating a light protein snack before you go to bed may help.

- The temperature in your sleeping quarters can affect the quality of your sleep, so make sure it is neither too hot nor too cold.

- Medications that are for sleep frequently cause sleep that is not favorable for creating a quality sleep pattern.

- Certain cheeses and deli meats (processed and smoked) can contribute to your open-eyed alter state when you are trying to sleep. Stay away from these meats and other hard cheeses because they contain an amino acid (tyramine) known to keep you alert: Parmesan,

Romano, and Asiago. Other foods that contain this amino acid are the fermented soy products such as soy sauce, tofu, and miso.

- If you are prone to heartburn or acid reflux, watch that you do not eat foods that give you this condition. Reduce or stay away from spicy and tomato-based foods at night. You want some sound sleep tonight, right?

Ch3: Critical Sleep Information to stop Insomnia

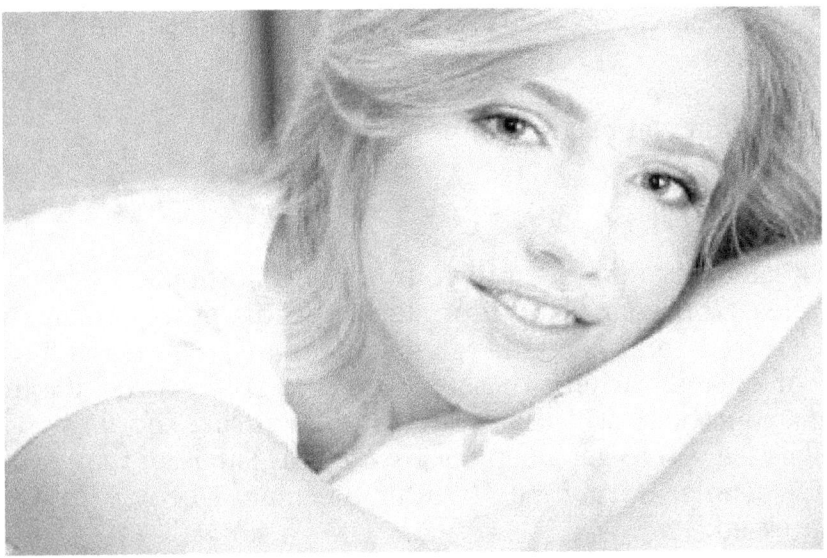

Deep Sleep

The 24-hour day cycle provides darkness and light to help you maintain a natural circadian rhythm. This rhythm activates all of your biological processes in your central nervous system, such as biological functions and cellular processes. These processes occur during the day, and during the night when you are asleep.

Without maintaining this natural circadian rhythm, which requires deep sleep, you will be susceptible to various detrimental diseases that can disrupt a good life and result in a shorting of life span.

One thing that is known, for sure, is that you need deep sleep, if you are to live a healthy life. So it is important for you to have a basic understanding about sleep. This will allow you to make changes, in your living patterns, so that you can get sleep you need.

When you wake up in the morning, do you feel invigorated and ready to face the day? Or, do you feel groggy and during the day you lack energy, even though you had more than 8 hours of sleep?

Here's what you need to know about sleep.

Melatonin

As it gets dark outside or in your home, a hormone, melatonin, is released preparing you for sleep. In this process, you start to get tired and sleepy. If you live in an area where you have a lot of overcast where the sun does not shine through often, then your body will release melatonin during the day. This will cause you to get sleepy or tired. This is one of the reasons why people during the winter become sleepy, tired, or depressed.

Sun Light

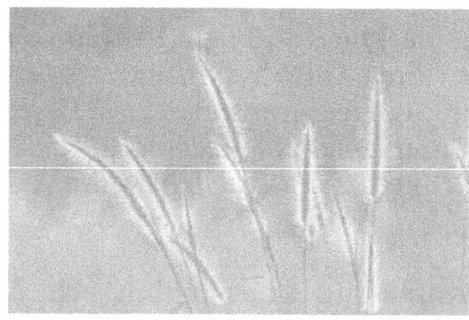

It is sun light that is one of the main factors that controls our sleep patterns. The lack of light or the intensity of light controls the release of a certain amount of melatonin. Each day you want to expose yourself to high levels of light, so that you don't produce melatonin during the day.

During the day, the sun will provide between 32,000 and 130,000 lux of direct sunlight. If you are not in direct sunlight you can get between 10,000 to 25,000 lux. Now, if your day is over cast you will get around 100 to 1000 lux exposure.

So how much light do you need during the day and how do you get it.

In Dr. Mercola's article, January 2014, called How the Cycles of Light and Darkness Affect Your Health and Wellbeing, he says,

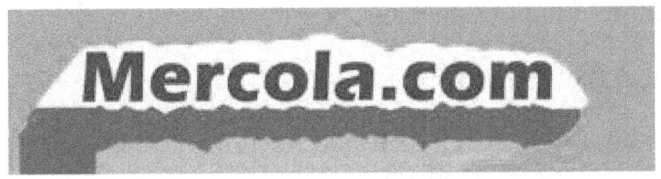

"Most people in Western societies spend the larger portion of each day indoors, which essentially puts you in a state of "light deficiency." In terms of light intensity, outdoor light is far more intense than indoor light." And he continues with a quote from Pardi,

" 'We're not getting enough bright light exposure during the day, and then in the evening, we're getting too much artificial light exposure. Both of those have the consequence of causing our rhythms to get out of sync.' "

Then, Dr. Mercola continues,

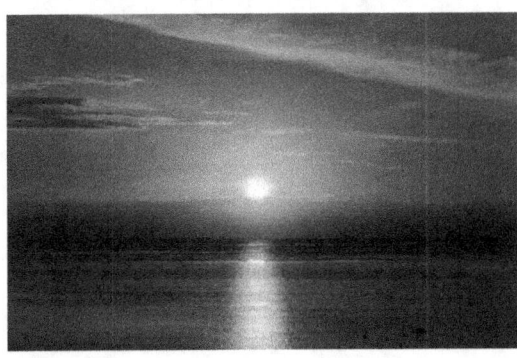

"So, in terms of practical advice to help you maintain healthy master clock timing, you want to get *bright light exposure* during the day. Many indoor environments simply aren't intense enough to

do the job well. So-called "anchor light" anchors your rhythm, causing it to be less fragile, so that light at night has less of an ability to shift your rhythm. As for how much light exposure you need, Pardi says *the first 30-60 minutes* of outdoor light exposure creates about 80 percent of the anchoring effect."

So, if it is practical for you, go outside for some activity in the morning sun or lunch time sun to get the sunlight, you can insure that proper amount of melatonin release during the night is not affected. Of course the amount of light you get before you go to sleep is also a factor.

Light You Need After Sun Down

It's not good to expose yourself intense light in the evening, since it limits the melatonin production.

As bed time approaches, you need to limit the amount of high intensity light you are exposed to. This starts your body producing melatonin, so that you get tired and sleepy.

When you are exposed to high-intensity light prior to bed time, your body produces less melatonin and you will not get a good sleep.

So, a few hours before bedtime, if your room has a high intensity, turn it off and use a low-intensity lamp. If you work on a computer or watch TV, stop watching one to two hours before going to bed.

In sleep research, it was found that even low intensity light during the evening can suppress melatonin release.

Even low intensity nighttime light has the capability of suppressing melatonin release.

Our eyes have special sensors that control when melatonin is released. When blue-light hits these sensors, melatonin is suppressed. You can produce melatonin by filtering out this blue light and fooling your body into thinking it is dark.

In an Internet article by Chris Kressler, called, How Artificial Light Is Wrecking Your Sleep, And What To Do About It, he says,

"So what's causing this epidemic of sleep disruption in our country? Many experts feel that our excessive use of communications technology (e.g. cell phones, laptops, television, etc.) is driving this significant level of sleep deprivation. If this is the case, it's no wonder so many Americans struggle with poor sleep, since 95% have reported using some type of electronics at least a few nights a week within the hour before bed."

Most electronic devices, including TV, emit a light at or close to the blue-light frequency. This is the frequency that blocks melatonin.

Lighting such as fluorescent light bulbs and LED lights has a high level of blue emissions. The regular incandescent light bulbs also emit some blue light, but it is much less than most florescent bulbs.

Here are three ways to overcome this blue-light effect.

First, you can avoid using these electronic devices 1 to 2 hours before bedtime. Sometimes this might not be possible because of your lifestyle.

Second you can use an amber tinted glass wear. This type of lens blocks the blue light. There are a variety of these types of light blocking glasses. You need to find a pair that works for you. Some people that use these types of glasses complain that it blocks too much light and makes it hard to see the computer screen.

You can check out these two Amazon pair:

Uvex-S1933X-Eyewear-SCT-Orange-Anti-Fog Solar-Shield-Fits-Over-Sunglasses-LENSES

Now, it you don't want to wear any type of blue light blocking glasses, you can stop using electronic devices, including TV, two hours before sleep. Or, consider using orange light bulbs.

Light Bulbs

Third, there are some light bulbs that you can buy that are coated to block off the blue light. Here is some information on this product, from the website,

https://www.lowbluelights.com/products.asp

Here is the description from their website page:

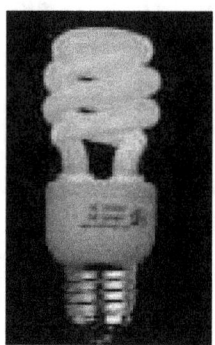

"This 120 VAC amber lamp (sometimes referred to as orange) has the light output of a 60 watt incandescent lamp and is suitable for low light areas such as nurseries and general background lighting. It has a coating that effectively removes the blue end of the spectrum. Its life is about 10,000 hours."

When You Sleep

Make sure you don't sleep with any light on in your room or any light coming into your room.

Body Temperature

Dr. H. Craig Heller, PhD, Professor OF Biology at Stanford University say that,

"When you go to sleep, your set point for body temperature - the temperature your brain is trying to achieve - goes down. Think of it as the internal thermostat."

So, as the time for you to go to bed approaches your body temperature starts to decrease. Being able to reach your body's temperature set point at night will determine how quickly you fall asleep and the quality of sleep you get.

When you get into bed, your body temperature needs to drop so that you can fall asleep. You can help your body reach its temperature set point by having the right room temperature. The cooler a room the easier you can fall asleep and reach a cooler body temperature during the night. If your room is too cold or too hot, you are likely to wake up during the night more than you should.

It is recommended that your room temperature be 64 to 70 degrees Fahrenheit. The temperature you need can be different for another person.

You have to experiment with different temperatures and sleeping with or without stocking or clothing to find the correct conditions that move your body into your right temperature set point.

When you wake up, your body temperature will increase, and this helps activate your body for your day's activities.

Himalayan Salt Crystal Lamps

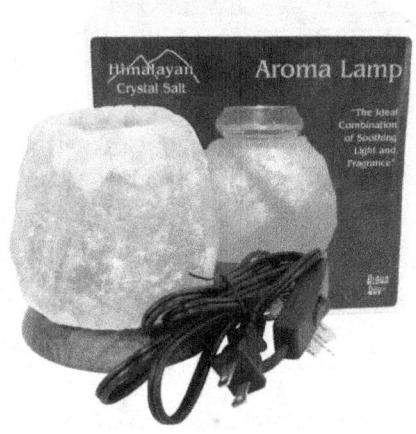

In the book, ***Himalayan Salt Crystal Lamps: For healing, harmony, and purification***, Clemence Lefevre answers the million-dollar question, "So what is a crystal salt lamp? It is a block of crystallized salt that has been carved out from the inside, leaving a hole into which a light bulb has been inserted. All you have to do is plug it in - the way you do a bedside lamp - for it to give off its soft, calming light. This light aids relaxation and meditation and also helps energize your whole body."

In his book, he describes how these soothing crystal lamps can protect you from the harmful electromagnetic waves from various electrical devices that are constantly bombarding you and interfere with sleep.

Besides being pretty, **salt crystal lamps** naturally emit the healing negative ions to rebalance the load of positive ions in the air by bonding with them and neutralizing their effects. These negative ions are very cleansing, can help reduce stress, provide health benefits for those that have allergies and sinus problems, and may help with situations of insomnia.

By putting the lamp in your bedroom and turning it on a few hours before sleep, the negative ions can help create a positive sleeping environment to help reduce insomnia.

Clemence Lefevre also points out that by having a salt lamp in your home,

"You can say good-bye forever to stress, recurring migraines, feelings of tiredness, insomnia, excessive nervousness, and lack of concentration. Thanks to crystal salt lamps your home will become a source of energy, dynamism, and vitality that will continuously regenerate you."

If the thought of having a little light on in your bedroom at night does not sound good, one trick is to have the lamp on a timer, so it can be on during the day hours and have it turn off shortly before your bed time. Or, just leave it on during the day and turn it off at night. if you think a salt crystal lamp might be for you, try it out.

Ch4: Sleep Stages You Need To Know About

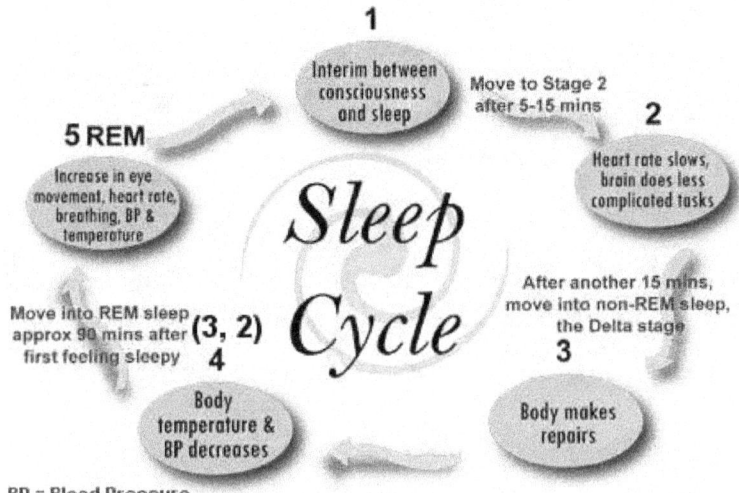

1
Interim between consciousness and sleep

Move to Stage 2 after 5-15 mins

2
Heart rate slows, brain does less complicated tasks

5 REM
Increase in eye movement, heart rate, breathing, BP & temperature

Sleep Cycle

Move into REM sleep approx 90 mins after first feeling sleepy **(3, 2) 4**

After another 15 mins, move into non-REM sleep, the Delta stage
3

Body temperature & BP decreases

Body makes repairs

BP = Blood Pressure

The Five Stages of Sleep

There are five stages of sleep and you move from one stage to the other naturally. You want the best deep sleep possible, and how long you stay in deep sleep depends on the many factors we have discussed earlier – light, blue light, temperature, and melatonin.

There are other factors that will produce deep sleep and these will be discussed later.

Hypothalamus

It is the hypothalamus that is responsible for maintaining and controlling your biological rhythms. These rhythms called circadian or diurnal, daily, rhythms, and monthly cycles are related to sleep, reproduction, or organ hormone excretions. There are hundreds of bodily functions that cycle during a 24-hour period.

During sleep, you cycle back and forth through 5 similar cycles. This cycling occurs 4 to 5 times. In each of these stages, your brain changes frequencies.

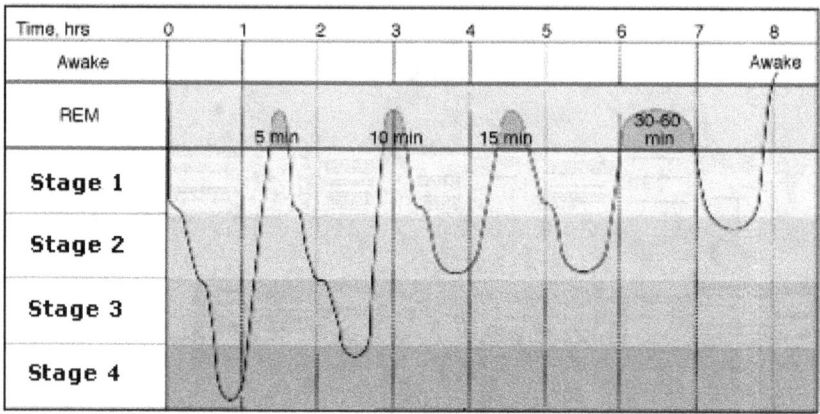

Stage 1

In the Stage One, you are moving from a wake state into sleep. Normally, you should fall asleep within 15 minutes. But, it takes 45 minutes for you to progress from stage 1 to 4. During this stage you can toss and turn.

In **Stage Two**, you move into a light sleep where heart rate and body temperature decrease.

Now, in **Stage Three**, your brainwaves start to change and slow down. In this stage, you move from a light sleep into a deep sleep. During deep sleep, your body is detoxifying and making body and cell repairs.

In **Stage Four**, you go into deeper sleep and it's this stage where you have the lowest brain waves. Your body is now in a cycle of making full repairs.

In **Stage Five**, you move back up to stage 1 in about 45 minutes. In the stage 1 position you move into REM sleep where you remain for about 10 minutes. During REM sleep your eyes move back and forth rapidly and heart rate and blood pressure increase.

It is during REM that you dream. During sleep you experience 3 to 4 REM periods. Each REM period is long than the previous.

Deep Sleep

Most of your deep sleep will occur in the first 4 to 5 hours of your 8 hours sleep. So the deeper sleep you experience, during the night, the less you need to sleep to feel good the following day. So to get the best sleep possible, you need to get to sleep within 15 to 20 minutes and cycle through the sleep cycles at least 3 times.

When you are young, your sleep time is around 7 to 8 hours. When you get older, 60 to 70, you sleep less, around 6 to 7 hours.

Older people sleep less because of the anxiety they have been holding back all their lives starts to surface during the sleep and causes them to wake up prematurely. Since they don't get their full sleep, they tend to nap during the day. When all their sleep is added up, they still end up sleeping around 7 to 8 hours per day.

Quality Deep Sleep

You want to get quality sleep and you get this by getting as much deep sleep as possible. When you lack deep sleep, you will not perform at your maximum potential, in all aspects, during the day.

Getting a lot of sleep doesn't mean good sleep, because you can sleep 8-10 hours and still feel tired during the day

Ch5: How Stress and Insomnia Are Killing You

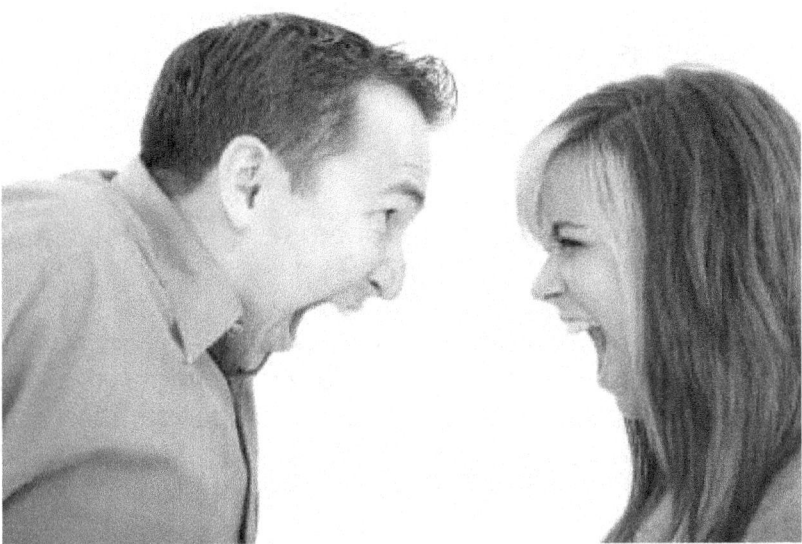

Chinese Medicine

In Chinese's medicine, each organ has an emotion associated with it. Your liver is associated with anger. If you harbor anger for a long time, this leads to an imbalance in your liver. If your liver is not balanced, then it can lead you to have anger. It's a cycle that can feed on itself.

Anger

If you are angry with someone, you need to find a way to resolve it or get past this. Keeping your anger for long periods or maintaining high levels of anger or hatred can affect your liver and result in illness and disease.

Anger can cause the lack of appetite, diarrhea, or indigestion. Suppressed anger can result in depression or menstrual disorders.

Studies have found that people who had high levels of hostility towards others have decreased immunity.

Fear and Letting Go

Your kidney is associated with fear. When some people experience a lot of fear, their bladder becomes uncontrollable, and they urinate. Children may wet the bed, when they are fearful.

Excess worry about life situations or problems can also weaken your kidney.

Your kidney and bladder are also related to "letting go of negative emotions." Since your kidney functions to remove un-needed body substances, it also works on eliminating bad or keeping good emotions. Your kidney has to balance everything that your body needs to keep healthy and to let go of that which is not.

Your kidney also works hard to keep your blood acid-alkaline balanced. You can see that keeping your kidney working properly will affect your skin's health.

Past Emotions

Usually, it is difficult to deal with the emotions that affect your liver, kidney, and bladder. These emotions are normally suppressed feeling, from your childhood or past that were never resolved and have been triggered by present interactions with other persons. Past suppressed emotions are a major force in the formation stress, anxiety, and illness.

In his book called, Why You Get Sick How You Get Well, 1996, Dr. Arthur Janov says that all sickness starts in your mind. In his years of practicing psychotherapy at The Primal Institute in Los Angeles, CA, he discovered how past traumatic

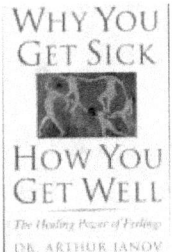

experience creates illness. Once the traumatic experience is relieved, the illness disappeared.

If you have anxiety, there are always some underlying emotions and feelings that are being expressed by your behavior.

Stress and anxiety are a representation of repressed traumas that you have experienced as a child or later in life. It can be an expression of those traumas, trying to burst out. Your body has a defense mechanism that holds back and buries past traumas.

Some effort has to be made on your part, to connect and release these traumas. Otherwise, as you clear your face, these suppressed traumas can move to some other part of your body, where they will be unseen and destroy tissue and body functions.

All past suppressed trauma that you have experienced has a representation in the body, internally or externally. This representation can be an internal body weakness or disease. Or, it can be a pleasant or unpleasant behavior. No matter how this suppressed trauma is expressed by your body, it plays a major part in your sleep patterns.

Your body protects you from early trauma that could have overwhelmed you, causing death or mental breakdown. It does this by suppressing the pain associated with the trauma. But, this suppressed pain is typically expressed by your body through distortions in your health, appearance or personality.

Daily Triggers

Past suppressed trauma remains hidden in your memory and throughout your body. The pain and suffering that you endured in the past is typically disconnected from your consciousness. This pain is usually triggered and brought into your consciousness by words, situations or events that occur in your present day's activities.

When your past pain is brought to consciousness, you will associate this pain with the interaction you are having with people in the present and not with past traumatic events. This is how you can become angry, hurt, or depressed more than what the present events call for.

Studies have shown that people with high stress tend to experience more anger, depression, anxiety, and suicidal feeling than those that do not.

If you find that you over react to various present day situations, you may want to consider working with some good therapists.

Psychological Therapy

Psychological therapy may be of help in resolving stress, anxiety, anger, and fear. Finding the right psychological process can be difficult, so if you have many emotional issues, this is the first place to start, for better sleep.

There is a psychological therapy, which addresses stress and anxiety that has been used successful during the last decade. It is called **Eye Movement Desensitization** and Reprocessing (EMDR). Developed by Francine Shapiro, Ph.D., it has been used with people suffering from traumatic incidences such as rape, sexual abuse, PTSD, anxiety, depression, grief, relationships, and eating disorders. To find the therapist nearest, you click the link above.

Tapes

Using hypnosis, affirmations, positive thinking, holosync tapes or hemisync tapes, or **paraliminal tapes**, can be some help, but it will not be a cure. These methods usually lead to continually suppression of your emotions, rather than providing a sort of cure. However, in combination with therapy, these tapes can be helpful.

Here are some titles to expect at the Paraliminal website. You can download them in digital form or order a cd.

- Sleep Deeply/Wake Refreshed

- Anxiety Free

- Letting Go

- Recover and reenergize

There are 38 different Paraliminal topics on personal improvement.

Meditation

Say the word "meditation" and in some people it conjures up images of monks sitting down and chanting "ommmm," but the truth is that meditation has many health benefits and is becoming one of the ways to treat chronic insomnia as well as other health afflictions.

It does not matter what religious affiliation you may have because meditation can be used to create what is called mindfulness. What is mindfulness you say? According to **Psychology Today**,

"Mindfulness is a state of active, open attention on the present. When you're mindful, you observe your thoughts and feelings from a distance, without judging them good or bad. Instead of letting your life pass you by, mindfulness means living in the moment and awakening to experience."

So what does this have to do with insomnia? Well, a lot of people who have insomnia also have what is called a mind full of thoughts that keep them awake into the night. Meditation can help pull the reins in on our random thoughts and help to calm us down and create an energy that will help us sleep.

You can buy one of the many meditation tapes that are available or follow these two simple steps right now as listed on the **Harvard Health Publications** web site and get started now:

Step 1: Choose a calming focus. Good examples are your breath, a sound ("Om"), a short prayer, a positive word (such as "relax" or "peace"), or a phrase ("breathing in calm, breathing out tension"; "I am relaxed"). If you choose a sound, repeat it aloud or silently as you inhale or exhale.

Step 2: Let go and relax. Don't worry about how you're doing. When you notice your mind has wandered, simply take a deep breath or say to yourself "thinking, thinking" and gently return your attention to your chosen focus.

Think of **meditation as the training** of the untrained mind and you will soon be sleeping like a baby.

Free Meditation Tapes
If you want to try some of the better free meditation tapes, head over to this site, **Mindful Muscle**, and get some unique Youtube mediations.

Ch6: How To Release Stress And Deal with Anxiety

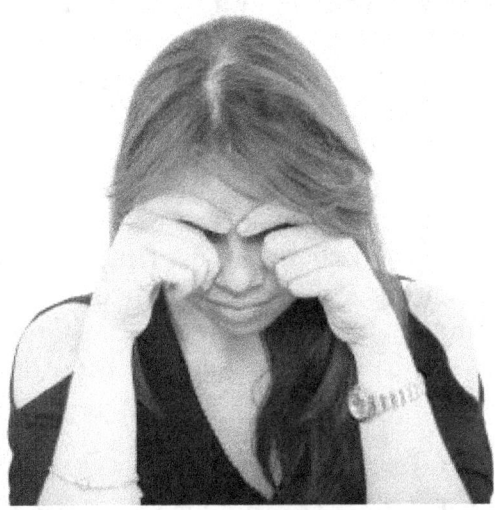

Even though heart and cancer kill more people than any other disease, anxiety and stress are really the number 1 killers. Without anxiety or stress fewer people would die of heart disease and cancer.

A Secret Therapists Use

In this chapter, you will discover information that is normally not revealed to you. This is done so that you may have a chance to have better emotional health, and of course, to get the sleep you need to keep you healthy.

This information is typically used by therapists who are afraid to tell you this since they feel you would not be able to handle your emotions. But your body has a build in defense system that will only allow you to feel those emotions that you are ready for. Of course, there are always some people that should be working with a therapist and not be using the technique outline here.

So read on to find a secret used by many therapists.

Anxiety Neurosis

Excessive anxiety is better known as **anxiety neurosis**. Anxiety is a condition where you worry about a specific or unknown thing, for a long time. Worrying for daily or short term things can be normal, but this still has some roots from unnecessary anxiety.

When you have anxiety neurosis, it can alter your sleep stages leaving you with a disturbed day. During the day, you can have headaches, sweating, difficulty concentrating, irritability, fatigue, nightmares, memory issues, or impotence. You frequently find it difficult to get along with others.

Past Traumas

In the past chapter, past trauma was discussed, and this is the source of anxiety neurosis. It is now well known that past childhood trauma and trauma encounter during adulthood leads to this neurosis. This occurs because these traumas were not allowed to go to completion, resulting in being buried in your nervous system and throughout your body in joints, muscles and organs.

These unresolved traumas need an external release, so they express themselves in the way you create a hectic and anxious lifestyle. The less trauma you have to deal with the calmer your life is, and you have no need to create a life with drama and situations that drain you of energy.

If you are not able to release all of your anxiety with your lifestyle, the excess will be dissipated internally. This release is energy that is destructive whether expressed in your unpleasant or pleasant behavior or whether expressed as some disease, such as a cardiovascular or cancer condition.

Reducing Anxiety and Stress

So, what can be done to reduce anxiety and stress? In the previous chapter various ideas given and when applied could reduce your stress, therapy, tapes, breathing, or mediation.

How Crying Reduces Anxiety

There is one other idea, crying, you know about, which can reduce your anxiety. However, you may not have being given the secret extension to crying, because crying can help you deal with stress, instead of expecting other to help you.

Anxiety and stress are pain. Crying relieves pain no matter whether it is physical or mental pain.

Women cry easier than men do. That is why they live longer. Crying has been looked down as a weakness, but the truth is crying gives you strength. When you are finished crying, you can see better what you need to do in your life. You have just given yourself stress relief.

Why You Cry

But, why do you cry? You cry because you have pain either physical or emotional pain. Physical pain is triggered by inflammation created by an external blow to the body or from a parasite attack from the inside of your body.

You cry from emotional pain because your internal suppressed pain received an external blow by someone saying or doing something that triggered your suppressed pain.

One-Step Beyond

You can use crying to help you relieve some of your suppressed pain. When you do this, you are going one step further than you normally do when you cry when someone has said something that hurt your feelings. However, you need to do this slowly, so that you don't get overwhelmed with feelings. When excess feelings start to surface, and you are not able to deal with them, then you need to see a therapist. But, for most people this may not be the case.

Crying is Triggered

Crying occurs when someone has triggered a feeling. You may feel that they don't care about or love you. You may feel they don't respect you. Or, they make you feel that they are better than you, or that they get more than you. But, whatever the feeling is it makes you cry.

How to Cry

Here's what to do. Find a place where you can cry without bothering people, a safe place. You don't have to cry in front of the people that hurt you, but that is ok if it happens. Remember that hurt and deal with it when you have some time during the day or evening.

Lie down and cry, if you can move into the hurt feeling right away. Cry about what happen or what was said to you to hurt you. As you cry for a time, now try to remember an incident from the past that was similar to why you are crying at the moment. It could have been a teacher, friend, brother, sister, relative or parent that made you feel the same way that you are crying about. Allow yourself to cry about this for a while. Cry as long as you need to this may be 30 minutes, an hour or even two hours. There is no time limit when you are hurting.

When crying your thoughts may wander, so what you can do is pick up with the new thought and see if it has some pain that you can feel. If not, go back to where the crying sensation is the most.

When You Finish Crying

When you finish crying like this, you will feel more relaxed and with less anxiety. Now, it can be that the feeling you're crying about may last for a few days or weeks. Just keep dealing with by crying.

You control your crying. Use it for anxiety and stress when you are triggered. It does not matter whether you are a woman or man. Crying is how your body deals with pain, and you need to help get rid of this pain by not blocking.

Once you start to use this crying tool to feel your present hurt and a little of your past trauma, your insomnia will start to decrease, and eventually it will no longer be an issue.

If you have nightmares, these nightmares may increase for a while, but this depends upon the intensity of your past trauma, since nightmares are an expression of your past trauma.

Crying and EMDR

EMDR was mentioned in the previous chapter and it's something you can add to your crying. EMDR is where you move your eyes left and right as you are into a feeling or are crying. What this does is as you cry you are accessing different parts of your brain for the feeling or pain you are experiencing. When you move your eyes back and forth you access the sound, light, image, touch, smell or taste of the feeling or memory you are crying about. This will make your crying more intense. In the beginning of using EMDR you may not notice a difference but the difference is occurring.

Ch7: Foods You Should Eat To Stop Insomnia

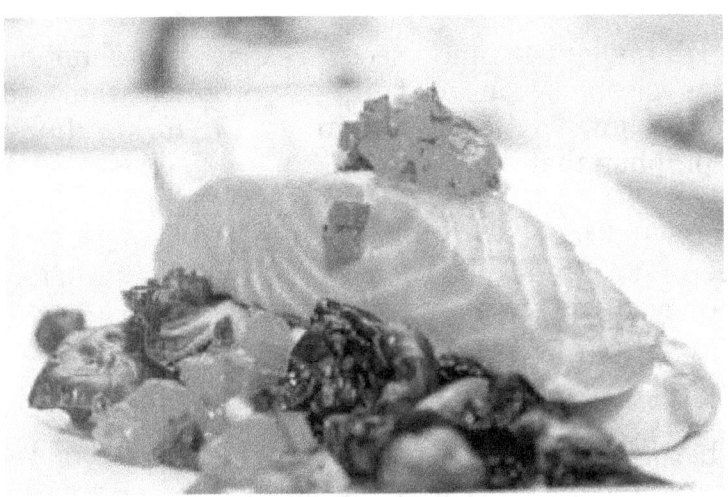

What to Eat

These are the foods that you can eat when you have insomnia. Eat foods that promote melatonin production like salmon, tuna or halibut, chia seeds, and fortified cereals. These foods are high in vitamin B6 (pyridoxine) which assists the body in making melatonin - the sleep hormone.

Another food that promotes melatonin production is miso soup.

Tryptophan

Bananas are a great sleep food as they not only contain vitamin B6, they also contain magnesium and potassium, which is needed for muscle relaxation as well as tryptophan which turns into the hormones, serotonin, and melatonin in the body.

Another tryptophan containing food is humus.

Foods with calcium help lower stressful feelings: plain unsweetened yogurt, milk, cheese also contains sleep-promoting tryptophan.

Whole-grains, nuts and seeds, especially almonds, can promote sleep because of the tryptophan they contain. Remember how you feel after eating a big turkey dinner? It's the tryptophan that is the relaxer.

Eating low-fat foods with little protein can help get you ready for sleep. Try a breakfast cereal without milk, fig bars, waffle with honey, or gingersnaps.

Herbal Teas

Many herbal teas have constituents useful to ease you to sleep. Try chamomile or a decaf green tea. Other relaxing teas are passionflower, hops, lemon balm, catnip.

Protein and Carbohydrates

Eating a bit of protein as a snack may help you sleep through the night: eggs

Oatmeal contains minerals such as calcium, magnesium, phosphorus, silicon, and potassium all of which can have a sleepy-time effect, and it is also rich in our friend melatonin. Remember to top off with some banana slices.

Honey

In her book, Food Your Miracle Medicine, Jean Carper makes this honey recommendation, "One of food's best sleeping pills is something sweet or starchy. Honey has long been used in folk medicine as a soporific. So, if falling asleep or staying asleep is a problem, try eating an ounce or so of sweet

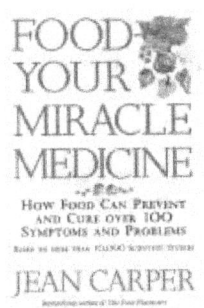

[pure honey]or starchy stuff about half an hour before going to bed. 'for most people this is an effective as a sleeping pill, but without the side effects of morning grogginess and the potential for abuse inherent in drugs'" says Judith Wurtman, Ph.D. a nutrition researcher at MIT an expert on the subject.

Milk

While milk chocolate may be a stimulant, which is not conducive to deep sleep, dark chocolate, on the other hand, contains tryptophan and magnesium. Only a small amount of chocolate is needed. This is a win for you chocolate-lovers!

Many people find a warm glass of milk can help fall asleep. Researchers don't believe in the glass of milk idea. But, some studies have found that milks contain natural opiates, which may contribute to better sleep. One possible way to use milk is to mix a warm glass of milk with a banana and a teaspoon of honey.

Honey and Citrus Juice

Here is a honey combination you can use before you go to bed. Add two teaspoons of dark honey to 1/2 glass of warm water. Then add the juice of one lemon or orange juice. You may want to adjust the amount of honey and juice to find the right combination for you.

Food for Stress

Here are some foods that you can eat throughout the day, which can help you reduce your stress by providing you with the chemicals your body needs to fight stress.

You need to eat complex carbohydrates, which help your brain make serotonin. Serotonin is a brain chemical that makes you feel good. Eat oatmeal, whole grains, brown rice or spelt.

Take folate which is a B vitamin and helps your brain process serotonin. You can get folate from black beans, spinach, cabbage, and asparagus.

Eat those foods that give you tryptophan such as crab, eggs, and shrimp. Tryptophan helps to create serotonin which in turn covers to melatonin.

Take vitamin C or eat those fruits and vegetables that are high in C. This vitamin is needed for your brain to make serotonin.

Coconut Oil

Coconut oil has been found to help regulate body functions that help sleep, when taken daily. In addition, this oil has been found to help reduce the effects of hypothyroism, which diminishes your energy and makes you feel tired.

Here's the amount of coconut oil you should be taking daily.

Body weight(lbs.)/tablespoon of coconut oil

- 175+/ 4 tbs.
- 150/ 3½ tbs.
- 125/ 3 tbs.
- 100/2½ tbs.
- 75/ 2 tbs.

Use only the pure cold-pressed virgin coconut oil designated as a dietary supplement. You can add it to your smoothies, salad dressings, or soups. There are many other ways to consume this oil, you just need to experiment.

Ch8: How Herbs Can Give You Quality Sleep

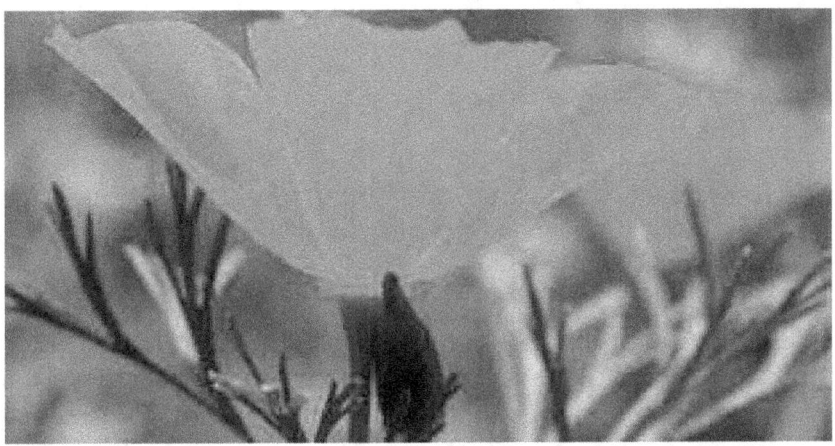

Herbs

Here are some herbs that you can use to relax and to reduce tension in your body. They are a great natural alternative to using narcotics or medical drugs. These herbs can help you with stress and anxiety, and these conditions typically relate to loss of quality sleep.

California Poppy (Eschscholzia California)

If you have access to the vibrantly colorful California poppy, you can make a tea out of the dried plant or extract. This plant contains alkaloids, which have a gentle sedative quality and can promote relaxation and support the nervous system. It is suitable for adults and children alike. Europe uses this herb with corydalis as a sleep aid. Combining it with passionflower will also help to bring on drowsiness.

Here's how to use it.

Drink up to 4 cups of this tea per day. Add one teaspoon California to one cup of hot water for 10 minutes. You can try finding dried leaves and flowers in a health-food store that carries dried herbs or look on the Internet. An extract may be the preferred method as the tea may be a bit bitter. Make sure you do not use this if you are pregnant, breastfeeding, or within two weeks of any surgeries.

Hops (Humulus lupulus)

Hops is another traditional and potent herb that is great for stress, insomnia, and nervousness. In addition, hops can lower your body's acid level.

WebMD states, "Some research suggests that taking a combination of hops extract plus valerian extract at bedtime helps some people fall asleep faster. It appears to take 28 days of treatment to see these benefits. However, a combination of valerian extract and hops extract seems to improve sleep quality similarly to bromazepam (Lexotanil) when taken for only 14 days."

This sounds like a good natural combo for fighting those sleepless nights. Other sleep-inducing combos include using hops with passionflower or lemon balm.

Although, hops is generally recognized as safe (GRAS), its sedative effects may increase certain pharmaceutical drugs, so check with your physician, if you are on any medications.

Jamaican Dogwood Extract

This is a powerful sedative and analgesic, which promotes a restful sleep for insomnia that is caused by pain, anxiety, or nervous tension. Its use is well-known in Caribbean medicine. The root bark of the Jamaica Dogwood is the part that has the anti-inflammatory, antispasmodic, and sedative properties. It is mostly taken in decoction form and may be combined with hops and valerian as listed on <u>Holistic online.com</u>. You can also find it prepared in tincture and in capsule form.

Improper use of Jamaica Dogwood can lead to side effects which may include gastric disturbances, nausea, sweating and numbness. Although not poisonous to humans, it could cause a heavy sedative effect if not used correctly. Use under the direction of a qualified healthcare practitioner as this herb can be potentially toxic. Do not use this herb if you are on other medications, pregnant, breastfeeding, or elderly.

Use 12 to 48 milligrams

Lemon Balm (Melissa officinalis)

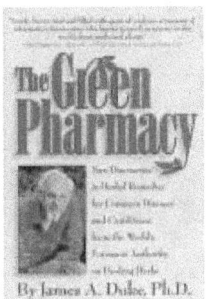

In his book called The Green Pharmacy, James A. Duke, Ph.D. recommends lemon balm for insomnia.

"Also known as Melissa, lemon balm is endorsed as both a sedative and stomach soother by Commission E, the body of scientists that advises the German government about herb safety and effectiveness.

The sedative action is attributed largely to a group of chemicals in the plant called terpenes. Several other herbs – juniper, ginger, basil, and clove – are better endowed with some of these chemicals, but none of them has the combination that lemon balm contains, and none of them has its reputation as a bedtime herb."

Lemon balm has a lemon-like smell and is part of the mint family. During the Middle Ages, it was commonly used as a calming agent. It can also be used alone or in combination with other herbs such as valerian, hops, and chamomile to promote sleep and soothe the nervous system.

Use lemon balm to ease your insomnia, if it is not too severe and comes from illness, indigestion or headaches. Use 1 – 2 cups of tea by adding two teaspoons of the dried leaf in hot water for 10 minutes. You can also use 300 – 400 mg in capsule form or in an extract.

Kava Kava (Piper methysticum)

Kava Kava is an excellent herbal remedy for calming moderate anxiety, stress, and insomnia. There are whole cultures that have embraced the Kava Kava plant and use it for a myriad of purposes. It is used medicinally and for ceremonial devotions of which they are very respectful towards the plant.

In a study listed on **PubMed.gov**, Kava Kava used alone or in conjunction with valerian root may be useful in the treatment of stress-induced insomnia.

Do not use this, if you are on medication, drink alcohol, or have liver problems. Always test out an herb to see what your reaction will be, when you take it, and check with your doctor if you are on medications.

Lavender (Lavandula angustifolia)

Lavender is effective in decreasing anxiety and promoting relaxation. It is also a powerful anti-bacterial and can work to balance hormones.

One way to utilize the powers of lavender is to inhale the essential oil. According to **www.everything-lavender.com**, "Studies have shown that when inhaled, individuals show a slowing of brain waves. This very clearly demonstrates the calming effects which in turn relieves stress from the individual as the body is brought into a more harmonious peaceful state."

I think this is something that everyone can use at one point or another, since we live in a stress-filled world. Lavender oil can be used to create a relaxed sense of mind and body. When properly applied, it can help to reduce your stress and depression levels. It has calming and relaxing properties, especially when inhaled.

Licorice Root (Glycyrrhiza glabra)

Licorice root can help you during stressful times. It also helps to normalize your blood sugar levels.

Excess stress can affect your adrenal glands and cause them to become exhausted which can contribute to bouts of insomnia. There are two types of licorice root: One that contains glycyrrhizinic acid which is its active ingredient and may cause side effects in persons with certain health issues. And one that has the glycyrrhizinic acid removed called deglycyrrhizinated licorice (DGL). DGL is used for persons who have specific health concerns, such as acid reflux or ulcers. Consult with your physician if you are on any medications before trying any licorice root products.

Red Clover Flower

It was the early American that discovered red clover was a good sleep remedy. Here how to use it.

Place two tablespoons of dried red clover into 8 oz. of hot water, for 10 minutes. Drain and add a touch of honey, then drink within 30 minutes before bedtime.

Valerian Root (valeriana officinalis)

A Valerian root is one of the most popular herbs for sleep and was even used in ancient times for insomnia and anxiety. It has been studied more than any other herb for various uses. It considered so safe you can drink a few cups per day to relieve stress, nervousness, or anxiety.

A special point about valerian is that it contains a substance called GABA (gamma aminobutyric acid) which is an inhibitory neurotransmitter that can promote sleep and calm the brain (*Natural Home Remedies for Insomnia* at **www.healthguidance.org**).

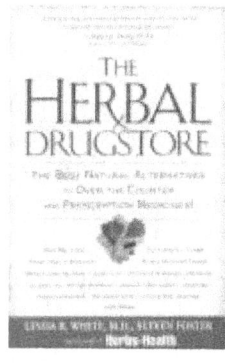

In her book, The Herbal Drugstore, Linda B White, M.D. talks about how to use valerian, "taken 30 to 45 minutes before bedtime: one 150 to 300-milligram capsule standardized to 0.8 percent valeric acid, or 300 to 400 milligrams in nonstadardized capsules...Valerian is not addictive, but if you're convinced you can't sleep without if, you could develop a psychological dependence. ... if this occurs stop using it."

When using valerian root for anxiety, you can take 450 mg up to three times a day. Be observant as to how you are feeling and reacting in order to know if the valerian root is helping you and not just making you. Do not take on an empty stomach.

Taking valerian root at higher doses (400mg – 900mg) about 30 minutes before bed causes the drowsiness needed for a good night's sleep.

Valerian and Lemon Balm

Now, there is a product that contains both **valerian and lemon balm**. this gives you the benefits of the two best sleep aids. you find this product called Valerian Extract with Lemon Balm by Prohealth

Passionflower (passiflora incarnate)

Although, not as strong as Valerian Root, Passionflower is an herb that has been used for hundreds of years against insomnia and is good for reducing muscle tension and for treating insomnia. And just like Valerian Root, it also contains the brain calming effects of GABA.

You can make a tea out of it before turning in for the night or you may take in extract or capsule form, if you prefer.

Sage (salvia officinalis)

Want to calm your mind? Try a cup of sage tea before going to sleep. You can use either the leaves (fresh or dried) and steep for a few minutes, strain, and drink. Not only is it a powerful antioxidant it is anti-inflammatory and soothing, so sleep can soon be on the way.

Using the oil of sage to calm your mind before sleep might also be helpful.

Chamomile (matricaria recutita)

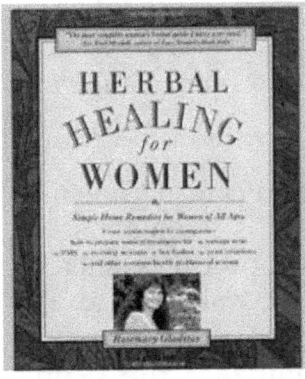

Chamomile is a natural remedy that is soothing, has anti-inflammatory and pain-relieving properties and is widely used in Europe. In her book, Herbal Healing for Women, Rosemary Gladstar states that, "Camomile is served in hospitals throughout Europe to calm and relax the patients, a practice I would like to see established in our medical facilities."

By drinking a cup of chamomile in the evening those soothing properties can calm your nerves and create drowsiness, so you can get to sleep.

Chamomile's sedative effects can be used for mild anxiety or nervousness because it has properties that will relax and calm you. This is an herb that can also benefit the health of your liver and lungs. It is considered a safe and non-toxic herb and is so gentle that you can even use it for children to help them calm down and go to sleep, as well as for colic and teething.

Chamomile has a pleasant taste as an herbal tea and may also be taken in capsule or extract form. As a sleep aid, you should take it about an hour before sleepy time.

Special note: Chamomile is related to the ragweed family, so if you have ragweed or daisy allergies, you may want to stay away from this particular herb. If you're pregnant, avoid Roman chamomile as this herb can cause miscarriage due to uterine contractions.

Wild Lettuce (Lactuca virosa)

Trouble sleeping? According to <u>International Business Times</u>, "Dr. Oz recommends you try taking 30 mg of wild lettuce extract before bedtime, the doctor wrote on his website. Also known as lettuce opium, the extract comes from the stems of the wild lettuce plant and has been shown in an animal study to have calming and sedative effects." And if you happen to have restless legs syndrome, it may be able to reduce and calm them.

Wild lettuce is a wild leafy looking plant and is also known by the names bitter lettuce or lettuce opium. It is the plant's sap, seeds, and leaves that are used in herbal products such as tinctures and extracts, teas, and capsules. Take 30 to 120 milligrams of the wild lettuce supplement before retiring. It may also be combined with valerian to enhance the sleepy-time effects.

When used for a short time in small amounts, wild lettuce can be a useful insomnia remedy. It is when it is used in a large amount, it can cause side effects like sweating, dizziness, rapid heartbeat, and difficulty breathing. Avoid if pregnant, breastfeeding, or if you have narrow-angle glaucoma, an enlarged prostate, impending surgery, or ragweed allergies. Always check with your healthcare provider before taking any herbs, especially if you are taking prescription drugs.

Using These Herbs

The best way to use these herbs is to buy them in half or one oz. packets and then, mix three or four of them in a one to one mixture, for example, one tablespoon of hops, one tablespoon of licorice root, one tablespoon of chamomile.

Boil this mixture, let it sit for 10 minutes, and drink it like a tea.

Here is an herbal mixture you can try that contains a variety of herbs that has help many people get better sleep. It's called **Revitalizing Sleep Formula** by Enzymatic Therapy and you can get it at Amazon.

All these herbs are wonderful natural remedies when used as teas, taken in capsules, or used in extract form. The thing to remember is before taking any herb or herbs in any form, please check with your physician for possible contraindications, especially if you are taking pharmaceutical drugs or have serious health issues.

Ch9: Special Insomnia Remedies That Produce Sleep

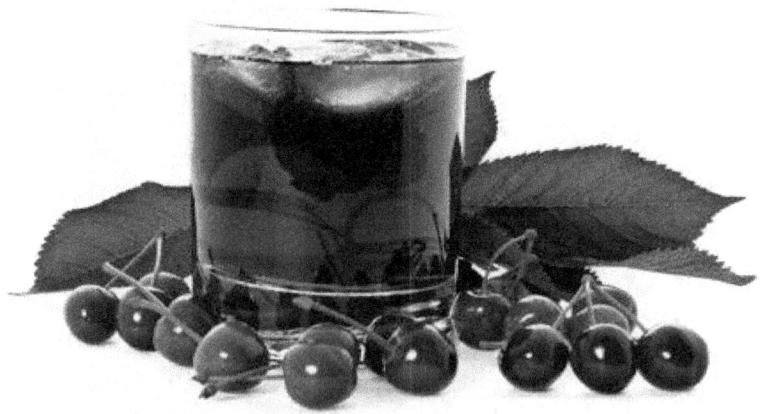

Here are some natural remedies that you need to use to get rid of your insomnia.

Cherry Juice

Cherry juice has found its way into the refrigerators of insomniac. This juice was found to give cherry drinkers longer and better sleep than those who did not drink this juice.

In a study from Northumbria University, UK, Montmorency cherry juice concentrate was found to provide 6-sulphatoxy melatonin, which promotes sleep. The subjects drank on glass upon waking and one glass before bed. This resulted in better quality sleep than those that did not drink the juice.

Fig-Dates

Here is another juice to consider before bed time, if you like dates and figs. This drink is high in sugar, so don't use if you have sugar issues. Mix in a blender a few figs and dates without pit, with some apple juice just enough to make a 8 oz. Drink an hour before bedtime.

Lettuce Juice

If you like making vegetable juices, here's what you can do. Juice some romaine or any other leafy green lettuce and add some apple juice to give it some flavor. Drink 1 hour before bedtime.

Passion Fruit juice

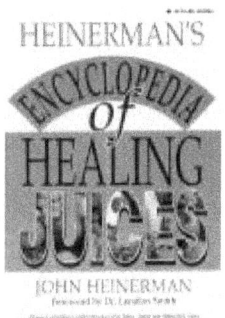 In his book called, Heinerman's Encyclopedia of Healing Juices, John Heinerman talks about, In Trinidad, the locals sell a bottled form of straight passion fruit juice, which they claim has terrific soporific [sleepy] effects. An doubts in the mind which the average tourist may have about this are quite literally, put to rest after a bottle or two of the stuff has been freely guzzled on an empty stomach. The person is usually out 'like a light' within half-an-hour..."

Here's where you can get pure **passion fruit concentrate**.

Poor Circulation

If you have poor circulation, you will have cold feet and hands. Just before bedtime, you blood vessels in your feet and hands expand to keep them warm. But, poor circulation keeps them cold and this can keep you awake. What you can try is to use different thickness stocks, to keep your feet warm. If you get your feet too warm, this may hamper your sleep.

Breathing Exercises

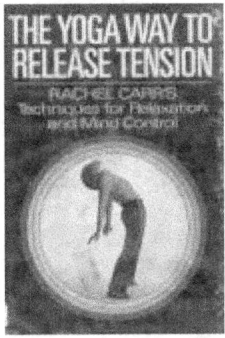

In her book, called The Yoga Way To Release Tension, Rachel Carr talks about how to breathe properly to get good sleep and to release tension.

"The purpose of Diaphragmatic Breathing is to stretch the lower lobes of the lungs with more air. This low, quiet breathing will calm emotions and induce restful sleep. It can be done either lying flat or sitting in a chair. Be sure to loosen your belt and collar. If you are sitting, place your hands limply on the thighs; spine straight but not rigid. If you are lying on your back, bend your knees with feet drawn to the buttocks and arms to your sides. It will help to place one hand on your abdomen and the other on your chest. The emphasis of breathing is on the abdomen. The chest is relaxed."

Then here is what Rachel says to do:

- Inhale deeply through the nostrils and expand the abdomen
- Exhale slowly through the nostrils while pulling in the abdomen to the back of the spine
- When you are able to control your breathing in this way, concentrate on maintaining a steady rhythmic pattern.
- Inhale to the count of 5 seconds
- Exhale to the count of 10 seconds"

Now, this is a simple technique you can do throughout the day. You can repeat this breathing 10 to 15 times a day. Try to be relaxed as you do this exercise. As you practice this type of breathing, your lung capacity will improve and you will release stress and anxiety.

When you do not breathe deeply or take short breathes as you breathe, you keep tension and anxiety inside your body, which creates damage throughout your body and prevents you from getting good night sleep.

Adrenal Exhaustion

If your life consists of a high-stress job or a situation where you are on the go all the time, your adrenals at some point will become exhausted. When this happens, you will feel tired, lack energy, and become less motivated. This condition will translate into poor sleeping patterns.

Here's what you can do to feed your adrenals the food that they need. Your adrenals need protein to create their hormones. When you are stressed or have low blood sugar, you use up a lot of your vitamin C. This vitamin is necessary to help make the adrenal hormones.

It's critical to replace vitamin C after stressful days, so after you eat a meal with protein, such as fish, meat, cheese, peas, beans, eggs, or nuts finish your meal with lemon, orange, or grapefruit juice. Or, you can just take 2000 to 4000 mg buffered vitamin C with a citrus juice without sugar.
In addition, to start regaining your adrenal power back, you need to sleep and sleep. Make it your priority to get more rest. Here's how to do it.

Get to bed at least one hour before you normally do and if you can't do this make sure you get to bed by 10 pm. Then get up at the time you normally do. Do this for a month to give your adrenal gland a chance to recover.

During your month of adrenal recovery, make sure you limit your exercises, since cortisol is released from your adrenal, when you exercise.

If you are looking for a supplement for your adrenal, you can checkout this product called **Adrenal Power Powder**.

Ch10: Natural Sleep Aids That Work Right Away

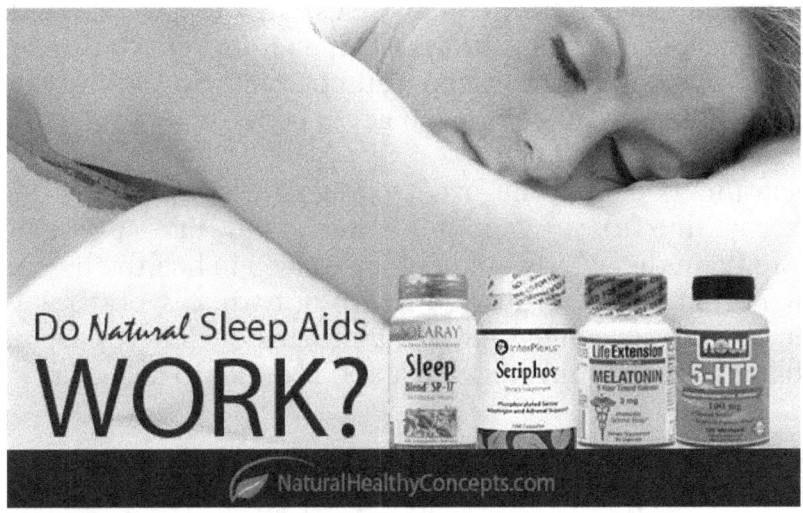

Ways to Get More Sleep.

For Men

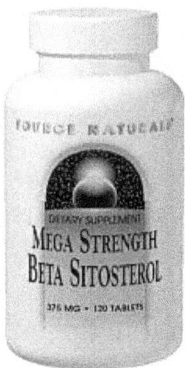

If you get up at night to urinate 2-3 times or wake up early in the morning to do this, you, mostly likely, have an enlarged prostrate. If your urination is weak or in spurts, this also indicates you have prostate issues. An enlarged prostrate will narrow your urinary track and not allow you to release all your urine from your bladder at one time. The result is you have to urinate frequently, during the night.

This will certainly have an impact on getting a good night sleep. Here is a supplement, <u>Mega Strength Beta Sitosterol</u>, that will help your eliminate frequent night urination and reduce weak and trickling urine.

Melatonin

<u>Melatonin is a natural hormone</u> released by your Pineal gland that regulates your sleep/wake cycles. As the day gets darker, your Pineal gland starts to release melatonin. If you wake up at night and can't get to sleep again or wake up too early, take 2-4 mg of melatonin before you get to bed.

Melatonin is commonly used to regulate sleep, adjust sleep patterns due to jet lag and travel, and may assist with insomnia in the elderly, and enhance sleep in healthy persons. Experiment with the dose to figure out what is best for you. You can purchase melatonin in sublingual or time release pills. Sublingual melatonin works fast and is easier to use.

Psychological Nutrients

The nutrients that are needed for psychological issues are,
- B vitamins
- Zinc
- Folic acid
- Selenium
- Chromium
- Omega-3
- Digestive enzymes
- Anti-oxidants
- 5 HTP

B Vitamins

The B vitamins are critical to many different brain functions.

5 HTP Supplements

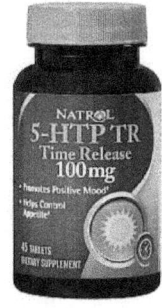

If you are plagued with depression, obesity, and craving carbohydrates, the supplement to take is 5 HTP. You want to make sure that you have some of these supplements in your diet.

D-Ribose

D-ribose is a sugar that is derived from blood glucose and is part of ATP molecule, which is stores and delivers energy to all of your cells. It is frequently used by body builders to take their workout to a higher level without muscle fatigue. If you are lacking energy, ribose is one nutrient that can give you additional energy.

Dr. Andrew Weil, M.D. says that,

"Ribose taken at the recommended dose is unlikely to do you any harm, but you should be aware that it is being added to many products, including energy drinks, and you may be getting more than you think. If ribose is working for you, you should limit your intake to no more than five grams three times a day."

It is better for you to take 5 gm. two times a day with food for sleep problems. Ribose is also good for fatigue, fibromyalgia, and heart disease.

Magnesium, Calcium and Vitamin D3

With magnesium, calcium and vitamin D3 in the same pill, you can reduce muscle and nerve tension. Always take D3 with your mag-cal supplement. D3 is need in this supplement in order for you to absorb the calcium. Here is where you can find this supplement with all three nutrients.

If you want to try only using magnesium without the calcium

or vitamin D3, the recommended product is called **Jigsaw Magnesium**, which contains added B6 and Folic acid. This magnesium will help you with leg cramps, stress, depression, and anxiety.

Sleep Tonight

Here is another supplement you can take called Sleep Tonight.

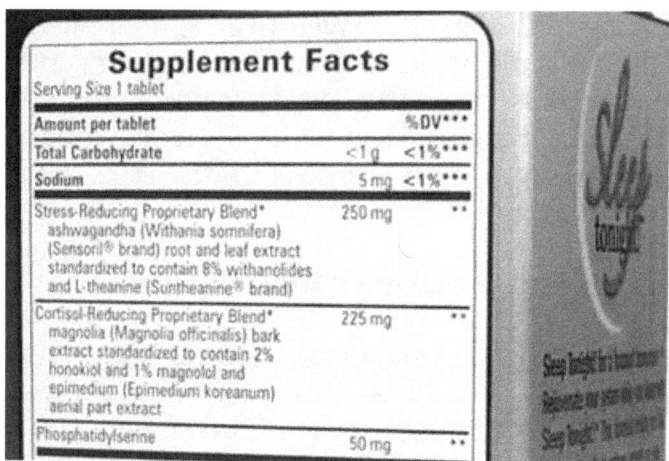

This compound produce by Enzymatic Therapy is designed for those whose mind continues to race once they hit their bed. This sleep product works by lowering your cortisol levels so that you are not in the stress mode. You can get this at iherb.com.

Suntheanine Is Stress Reducing

Suntheanine is the trade name for Taiyo that contains the pure form of the amino acid L- theanine. This amino acid, which is found in green tea, produces alpha waves that help you relax.

In addition, it helps in the production of GABA, which is needed for sleep.

Use 50 – 200 mg just before sleep, with 400 to 600 mg of magnesium.   Or, take it with the Calcium, Magnesium, Vitamin D complex.

If you buy L- theanine in another brand, make sure the use the pure form of L – theanine in the formulation.

Ch11: How To Do Exercises That Help You Sleep

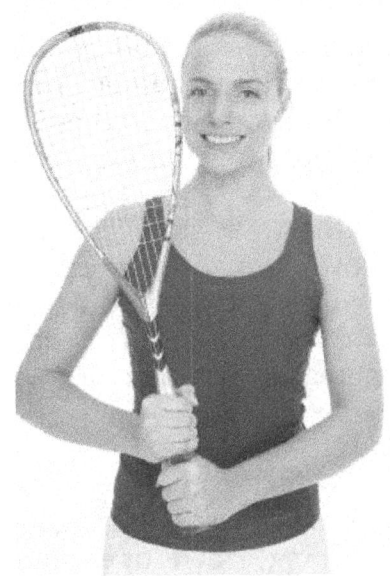

Exercise for Quality Sleep

In a study about exercise and sleep reported by researchers in the *Journal of Clinical sleep Medicine*, they found that people who exercise regularly fell asleep 55 percent faster and had a 30 percent decrease in the time they were awake at night.

Various exercises will provide you stress relief, by releasing endorphins. Doing frequent exercises, will help you manage your anxiety and stress. Practicing Yoga is effective in reducing stress. But, this is true of the many other exercises you might do.

One of the best ways to exercise is to do "interval exercise." In this process, you exercise fast in a short burst followed by a slower pace exercise or rest period and then again, a fast burst.

Studies have shown that interval training will help you become healthier than the typical lengthy steady exercises – treadmill, aerobics, bike riding, swimming, etc.

Walking

So what are the exercises you should be doing? There is no need to go to the gym and spend an hour running on the tread mill or riding a bike. Sure you can do these exercises, but they are not the best ones to lose weight.

If you want to walk, the walk as quickly as you can for one minute, then walk slowly until your heart rate comes back to normal, then walk real fast again. Rotate from fast to slow walk for about 5 to 6 times. You can increase these frequencies as you increase your stamina.

Other Exercises

There are many other exercises that are good for you. If you play sports and like riding a bike or swimming, then this is what you should do. Doing yoga is also an excellent exercise or dancing. You pick the exercise you like to do so.

If you walk, walk for a comfortable distance and then either try to increase your walk every day. Or, you can walk the same distance, but walk it faster.

Rebounder

Using a rebounder is another way to exercise at home. With the rebounder you can jump up and down and help tone your muscles. In addition, you activate the lymph liquid in your body to circulate better. This is an excellent way to help your body detoxify, especially if you do this in the morning.

Actually, doing your exercise in the morning will definitely help your body detoxify and help you lose more weight.

The Pace Program

There is another program that is one of the best ways to exercise. It is called the "PACE" exercise program. You can learn more about this on the Internet. This program is great for and for strengthening muscles, getting rid of stress, and losing weight. It is designed to build up your cardiovascular system and make you fit. The Pace program shows you how to do Interval Exercise which is the type of exercise you should be doing to build up your health and get better sleep.

Ch12: Insomnia Plan That Will Change Your Life

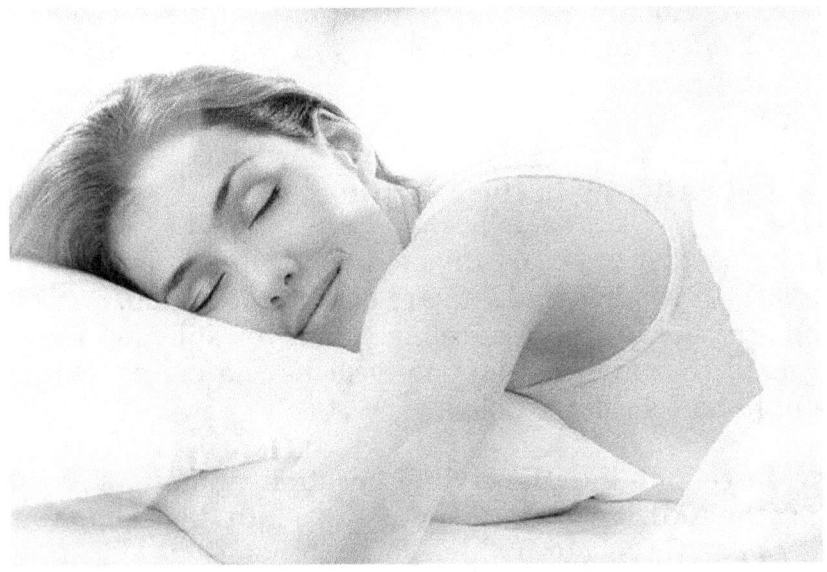

Insomnia can turn into a serious condition, which can lead to other diseases, because of nutritional deficiency. Here is a plan for you to start out with, so that you can reduce and eliminate your insomnia.

Short Period of Insomnia

In most cases of insomnia that last for a few days, you will get over it by yourself. But, if you have continual insomnia, then using the remedies and supplements listed in this book, you will help you eliminate your sleeplessness quickly.

If you lose sleep for a couple of days, from being worried about some upcoming event, this is not a big problem. This will pass, but if you continue having sleeping problems, here are some things you can try.

If you have started to use drugs for insomnia, then this program will not help you. It is best not to use any medication for sleep, if you want to use this program.

There are nine different areas that you can make changes to that will affect the sleep you get. Try to make a change in each of these areas, so you will have a better chance of creating great sleep.

1. First Thing in the Morning

When you first wake up, this is a good time to examine how you feel. If you had a nightmare or a crying dream, then it's a good time to work on this feeling. Or, if you still have a feeling triggered the previous day and still have a crying sensation about it, here's what to do.

Let yourself fall into the crying sensation, and as you do start doing the EMDR eye movement. Move into the feeling even if it's not deep crying or if only a few tear come out of your eyes. When you finish you are ready to get up. Do this for 10 to 30 minutes, so that you can discover how to do it better. Don't give up if nothing is happening.

First, drink a glass of water with the juice of one lemon. Now, it's time to get some morning sunshine. Take a walk outside for 20 to 30 minutes. If you prefer, you can get your sunshine during your lunch hours.

If you exercise, this is a good time also. You can exercise after or before your walk. Whether, you exercise in the morning or afternoon is up to you. You have to determine when you have the time and energy to do your exercise.

2. Meditation

Find 30 minutes when you will be free and not disturbed. Use this time to listen to relaxation or mediation tapes – holosync, Paraliminal, or meditation tapes.

3. Morning Breakfast

For breakfast, you can eat a light protein meal, but rotate it with a fruit and fruit and vegetable juice breakfast every other day. Use unprocessed oatmeal frequently with banana, raisins and other fruit toppings. Look over the section in chapter 2 called *"Miscellaneous Causes for Insomnia"* and apply some of these principles.

4. Day Time Light

Make sure you get plenty of day time sunlight. You can get sunlight through a window at home or office. Florescent light is not the light you need. This light has a narrow band of frequencies and tends to disturb your circadian cycle. In addition, they flicker on and off because the power it uses pulsates. This pulsing causes untold health issues. You can compensate for living under florescent lighting by getting as much sunlight as possible, during the day. Use incandescent lighting when possible, it has a broader light frequency than florescent.

5. Foods to eat during the day

Check the chapter on food to eat. You will want to eat those foods that have L- tryptophan – fish, seeds, cereals, humus, yogurt, cheese, whole grains, nuts, figs fruit, and vegetables.

6. Lighting before bed time

About an hour before bedtime, start to dim your lights and only have a yellow or small wattage incandescent light on. If you have a salt crystal lamp now is the time to turn it on. Try not to watch TV or work on a computer during this hour.

7. Herbs to drink before bedtime

There are many different herbal teas to drink before bedtime, and you need to experiment with different ones to see which ones work for you. Here is a list of some of them. Use a bit of honey to sweeten them.

- Chamomile
- Hops
- Hops and valerian extract
- Lavender
- Licorice root
- Jamaican Dogwood extract
- Kava kava
- Lemon balm
- Passionflower
- Sage
- Valerian
- Valerian and Lemon Balm
- Wild Lettuce

If you want a package sleep formulation, use this in place of teas and see if they work for you – Sleep Tonight or Suntheanine.

8. Special Insomnia remedies

- Drink cherry juice in the morning day or evening. Use a juice concentration and dilute with water to your liking.

- Blend a few fig and dates with apple juice and drink just before bed. You can also just try eating a few figs in season.

- A diluted or passion fruit extract

- A glass of milk with banana and honey

- Eating a large meal before bed diverts all your energy to digestion inviting insomnia. This is not a time when you want that to be happening, so if you must eat before bed choose a light protein snack which will keep your blood sugar balanced and will help you sleep.

- Drinking liquids before bed may interrupt your sleep by causing night time urination. Drink all your liquids from 2-3 hours before bedtime.

9. Supplements to use before bedtime

- There are many different supplements to take, so you may want to choose only a few as you start this program and then add more as time goes on.

- For men, use Beta Sitosterol for frequent urination at night.

- Take melatonin and start with a small dose. Start with .5 mg or 1 mg. If you don't have any side effects, or if it doesn't do anything for your sleep, you can add 1 mg until you reach 6 mg.

- Take B-50 or B-100 and add to this fish oil, digestive enzymes, and selenium.

- If you are bothered with depression or are trying to lose weight use 5 HTP.

- Always take magnesium, calcium and vitamin D3 during the day after your lunch.

10.   Exercise to do

- Exercise is a must for this program. Take daily walks for sunshine. Then do any exercise you like and try out the Pace Exercise Program. Yoga is another exercise that is great for anxiety and stress.

11. How to get quality sleep

- Follow a sleep schedule where you go to sleep at the same time every night and awake at the same time every morning. This can contribute to you getting a good night's rest.

- Do something calming before sleep like reading a book on the couch without any distractions: TV, computer, or phones. Put on some relaxing and calming music to soothe your body.

- Taking a hot relaxing bath a couple of hours before sleep can do wonders for bringing on a restful sleep.

- When bedtime is close, limit your exposure to blue light that comes from your lighting, TV, computers and other held hand devices.

- Keep your bedroom perfectly dark. Don't sleep with any lights on.

- If you sleep with an air conditioner or heater system, keep your room between 64 to 70 degrees Fahrenheit. You may have to experiment to find the right sleep temperature.

- Keep a salt crystal lamp in your bedroom so as you prepare for bed you aren't exposed to the harsh normal lighting.

- Keep your night clothing loose. Tight clothing will interfere with your sleep cycles.

- Keep your feet warn at night, if you have cold feet.

12. Dealing with stress and anxiety

- Using a variety of different meditation and holosnyc tapes will help you with stress. Use these daily.

- By using yoga or other types of exercise this can decrease you tension, stress, anxiety.

- You can use crying and EMDR, when you are triggered by daily interactions with people. This is one of the best ways to reduce anxiety and stress. Don't believe that crying is not good for you. It's the only way your body has to feel your present and past pain.

There you have it. A program you can follow. To start with do a little from each of the twelve steps and more as time passes. Don't get stress or anxious about using this program. Just ease into it, even by doing one step at a time.

Ch13: Author Information

Rudy Silva is a natural consultant nutritionist educated in the United State in Nutrition and Physics. He is a graduate from the San Jose State University in California. He is author of 30 other e-books on natural remedies. He has authored a newsletter in natural remedies for over 4 years. He has many websites promoting special recommended products and information.

For more natural remedy books that can help you, go now to this site:

http://www.amazon.com/Rudy-Silva/e/B00572F5SS

Rudy Silva is a natural consultant nutritionist educated in the United State in Nutrition and Physics. He is a graduate from the San Jose State University in California. He is author of 30 other e-books on natural remedies. He has authored a newsletter in natural remedies for over 4 years. He has many websites promoting special recommended products and information.

Give A Review

And, don't forget to give a review for this e-book at Amazon. It's not hard to give a review. It can be only a sentence or two. You don't have to leave a long review. A short review helps other people decide if they want to buy a book. So give a short review and give your thoughts to help other people and to help the author improve his book.

http://www.amazon.com/Rudy-Silva/e/B00572F5SS

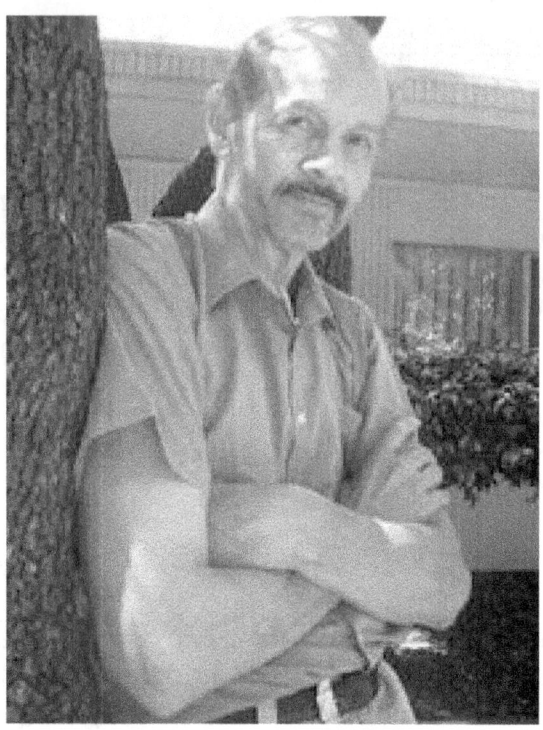

To you, creating better health and more happiness,

Rudy S Silva

www.ingramcontent.com/pod-product-compliance
Lightning Source LLC
Chambersburg PA
CBHW070603290526
45790CB00002B/759